GIFTING
BATHBOMBS

Project Book

Learn how to make a collection
of colourful bath bombs,
perfect for gifting

10 projects inside

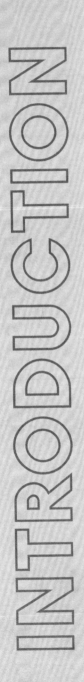

INTRODUCTION

Everybody loves a good pamper and long relaxing bath at the end of the day, so what better way to fully indulge than creating your own, personalised bath bombs.

In this book you'll find everything you need to get you started on your very own bath bomb journey.

We've included a number of recipes with different shapes, colours and scents!

Our recipes are designed to be easy to follow so you can be confident of making the perfect bath bomb, whether you're brand new to bath bomb making or a professional!

We've included everything you'll need to make your very own heart shaped bath bomb, the perfect gift for a loved one, or even for a present to yourself.

All the additional ingredients and equipment are readily available so you should have no problem getting everything you need.

KIT CONTENTS

WHAT'S INCLUDED:

- Bath powder mixture
- Purple dye & bicarbonate of soda mix
- Heart shape bath bomb mould

WHAT YOU'LL NEED:

- A large mixing bowl
- A teaspoon
- A wooden stirrer
- Gloves
- A dash of oil , vegetable, coconut or essential oils (we'll go onto the essential oils a bit later on)
- Cling film
- Scales (optional)

Below you'll find some handy tips to help you along your bath bomb journey. You can refer back to these for all the projects in this book...

TIP 1: MOISTURE IS IMPORTANT

Too little moisture in the bath bomb mix and it won't hold together. Too much moisture and the bath bomb will never come out of the mould. Use a teaspoon to add a small amount of moisture (water) at a time.

TIP 2: MORE IS BETTER THAN LESS

When filling the moulds you want to make sure you have enough bath bomb mixture. You want to slightly overfill and press together firmly.

TIP 3: TAP THE MOULDS

Do not twist the mould as this may cause the bath bomb to crumble. Try lightly tapping the mould on the table a few times before gently pulling the mould apart.

TIP 4: YOUR BATH BOMB WORKSPACE

To reduce mess, work in a space that is easy to wipe down and clean. We also suggest working in a space where the bath bombs can be left to dry for 24 hours.

TOP TIPS

TIP 5: WHAT COLOURING TO USE

Make sure you use water soluble colouring, specifically made for bath bombs. Gel colouring won't spread evenly.

TIP 6: SPEED IS KEY

Once you've added any liquid to your mixture, you need to work quickly to mix everything together, this will stop it from drying out before it's formed.

TIP 7: HOMEMADE MOULDS

You can use almost any shape to create a bath bomb mould, why not try yoghurt pots, silicone ice cube trays or silicone cupcake trays – just be sure to use a material you can easily remove the bomb from.

TIP 8: WHERE TO LEAVE YOUR BOMBS

Be sure to leave your bath bombs on a flat surface and in a non-humid environment.

TIP 9: DO NOT BE AFRAID TO START AGAIN

If your mixture isn't sticking together and you can't form the shape in your mould, then put it back in your bowl and start again. If you've added too much moisture then leave it in the bowl to dry before mixing again.

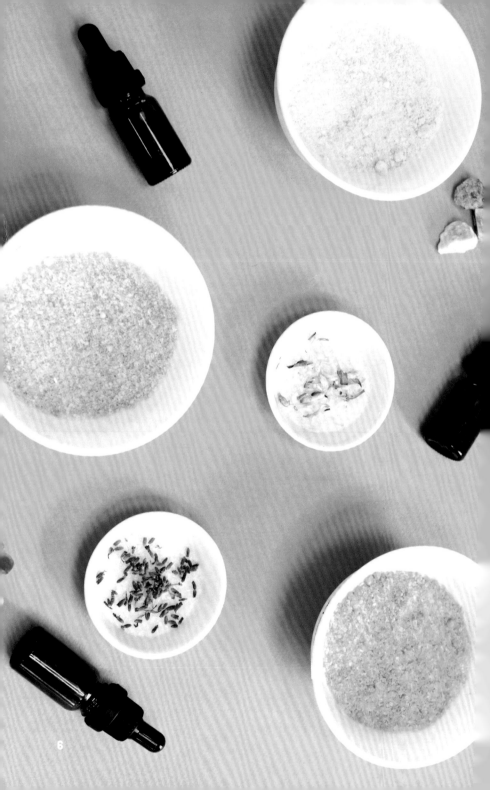

A GUIDE TO ESSENTIAL OILS:

Formed from plants, flowers and seeds, essential oils have a number of benefits from mental to physical health. As well as being known as a great stimulus to the brain (we'll cover in what ways on the next page), they smell amazing and are the perfect addition to any bath bomb.

Alongside smelling great and helping to relax or invigorate you, bath bombs work as a great moisturiser for the skin.

We recommend you test your essential oils before using them. A good way to do this is to add a few drops into a moisturiser and rub onto the back of your hand. As well as checking you like the smell, it's also a good way of testing for any allergies – remember these are natural oils and everyone reacts differently!

WARNINGS:

All the makes included in this book are designed for adults and are not suitable for children under the age of 14. Keep all ingredients and finished products out of the reach of children.

Some ingredients may irritate; always avoid contact with eyes. If ingredients come into contact with eyes or skin, wash with cold water immediately.

Wear gloves when handling the bath bombs to avoid irritation.

Do not ingest; if accidentally ingested drink water and seek medical advice.

When handling the melted oils, ensure these are cool enough before touching.

If pregnant or under the age of 10, be careful when selecting essential oils and the quantities used.

We recommend wearing old clothes or overalls and covering your work surface. Pigment in product may stain (can normally be removed with a household cleaner).

LAVENDER

This must-have oil is a favourite for a reason. It promotes calmness, relaxes muscles and is used to aid sleep.

PEPPERMINT

Refreshing and cooling, peppermint's powerful smell can invigorate and sharpen the senses. It is also good to soothe irritation.

TEA TREE

Harvested from the leaves of the tea tree plant, this popular essential oil has been used for centuries to help sooth the skin.

CHAMOMILE

Chamomile is a herb, that comes from a daisy-like flower. Its silky texture leaves the skin feeling healthy and refreshed.

ROSEMARY

This beautifully fragrant oil is regularly used in spa products and will leave the whole house smelling distinctively fresh and clean.

CINNAMON

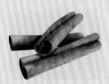

With its sweet and spicy scent, Cinnamon is used in aromatherapy for its mood enhancing and relaxing properties.

GINGER

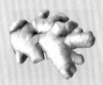

Ginger comes from a small root but packs a big punch. This zingy essential oil is said to have stimulating properties that promotes healthy skin.

LEMON

Lemon essential oil is a completely natural ingredient that is made by extracting the peel from fresh lemons. Lemon oil will leave you feeling clean, zesty and energised.

ROSE

Boasting a wonderful romantic scent, rose oil is a gentle moisturiser and wonderful toner for the skin.

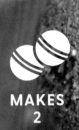

MAKES
2

HEART
BATH
BOMB

HEART BATH BOMB

The perfect shape to give to a loved one, or maybe even treat yourself, fizzy and purple it's sure to add some sparkle to bath time! We have included everything you need to get started with this bath bomb.

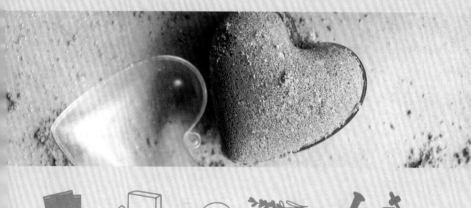

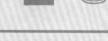

YOU WILL NEED

· A mixing bowl (similar size to a large microwavable jug)
· A teaspoon
· A wooden stirrer
· Gloves
· A dash of oil, vegetable, coconut or essential oils
· Cling film
· Scales (optional)

KIT CONTENTS

· Bath powder mixture
· Dye & bicarb of soda mix
· Heart bath bomb mould

METHOD

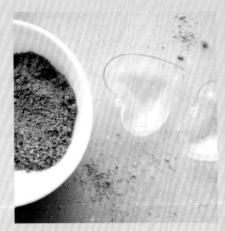

1 You'll want to start by preparing your workspace and laying out your materials. Make sure you have a clean, tidy space to work in. It is best to have an old cloth ready for any spillages.

2 It's also a good idea to tear a piece of clingfilm approximately 20-30cm long, so you're ready for later in the process.

3 Put on your gloves and gently open the bath bomb mixture, be careful not to inhale the powder.

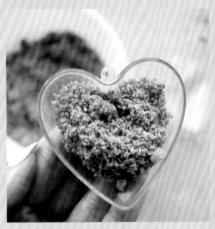

4 Pour half of the bath bomb mixture directly into the mixing bowl.

5 Take the purple bicarbonate of soda powder and add half of this into the bowl with the bath bomb mixture.

6 Stir the contents of the bowl together until it's well mixed.

7 It's time to add the moisture to your bath bomb mixture. If you'd like the bath bomb to have a fragrance, use an essential oil of your choice. Look back at our essential oil guide at the beginning of the book to select the fragrance that's best for you. Add one teaspoon and stir well. Alternatively, for a non-scented bath bomb, use an oil like vegetable or coconut and add one teaspoon.

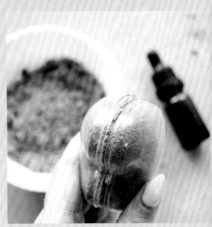

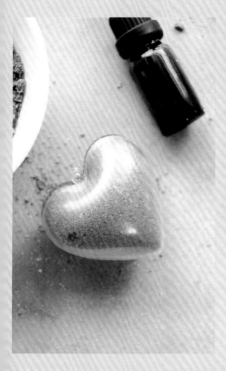

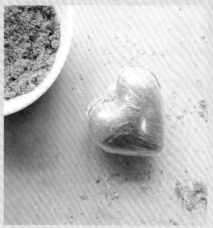

11 Place your two mould halves together and press the mould for 10-15 seconds. Do not twist or move the moulds once joined as this will make it harder for them to combine and could break the mixture.

8 Now it's time to add water, start by adding half a teaspoon to the mixture first of all. You are looking for a consistency similar to wet sand. Stir well and quickly once the water is added. When you add the water, the mixture will start to fizz but don't worry this is ok!

9 Now it's time to start filling the mould. Remember it's key to move quick at this point to avoid the mixture drying out.

10 Compact your moulds so the mixture fills just above the rim of the mould. We'd recommend filling just over the top of the mould but don't press it down. Leave the mixture on the top loose.

12 Wrap your moulds tightly in cling film 2- 3 times. This will stop moisture getting to them whilst they set and ensure the perfect bath bomb.

13 Set aside the wrapped bath bomb and leave overnight in a non-humid area.

14 The next day, carefully remove the bath bomb from the moulds. To remove the bath bomb, do not twist the mould as this may cause the bath bomb to crumble. Try lightly tapping the mould on the table a few times before gentling pulling the mould apart. Ta da!

15 Run yourself a bath, pop your bath bomb in and enjoy!

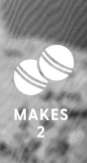

MAKES
2

RASPBERRY

RASPBERRY

What's better than the smell of fresh berries in the summer?
Why not re-create that with your very own raspberry bath
bomb!

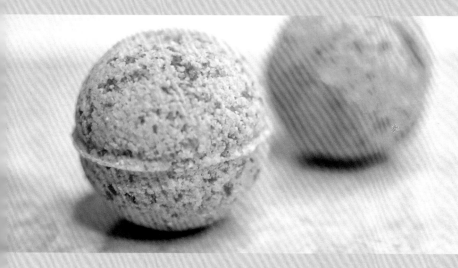

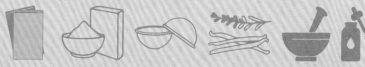

YOU WILL NEED

· A large mixing bowl
· A small mixing bowl
· Microwave
· Microwavable mug
· Whisk
· 2 x bath bomb moulds
· Cling film

INGREDIENTS

· Bicarbonate of soda 100g
· Cream of tartar 25g
· Corn starch 50g
· Epsom salt 2 tbsp
· Raspberry essential oil
  6-8 drops
· Coconut oil 1 – 2 tbsp
· Pink & red colouring
  5-10 drops

METHOD

1 Always refer back to your first bath bomb and make sure you've got your work surface ready and all your equipment to hand.

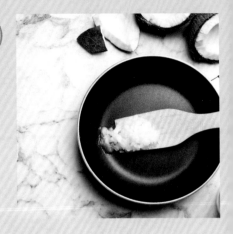

2 Take your microwavable mug and add 1 – 2 tablespoons of coconut oil, 5 drops of your pink colouring and 6 – 8 drops of your raspberry essential oil.

3 Microwave for 60 – 90 seconds or until the mixture is completely liquified. Make sure to only microwave 20 seconds at a time so you can check on progress. This is your oil base.

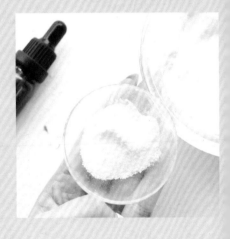

4 In your small bowl, add 1 tablespoon of Epsom salt and 8 drops of red colourant, stir thoroughly.

5 In your large mixing bowl, add the bicarbonate of soda, cream of tartar, corn starch and Epsom salt before mixing thoroughly.

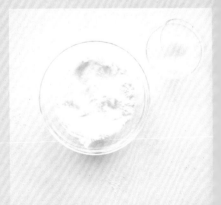

6 Pour your liquid mixture into the bowl of dry ingredients. We suggest doing this slowly whilst whisking throughout.

7 Add a teaspoon of water to your mixture and stir again.

8 Once the two mixtures are combined, give it a mix with your hands to ensure it's all mixed together, you don't want any lumps.

9 It's time to add your small mixing bowl of red colouring & Epsom salt. Ensure this is fully whisked through so you get an even colouring.

10 You are looking for the wet sand consistency again. Refer back to the tips page for how to achieve this.

11 Start to compact your bath bomb moulds and fill again just above the rim - the same as you did in your first project.

12 Place your moulds together and hold for 10 - 15 seconds. Wrap in clingfilm and leave overnight.

13 Leave overnight in a non-humid place and remove from the moulds the next day.

14 Wrap in some tissue for a lovely homemade gift!

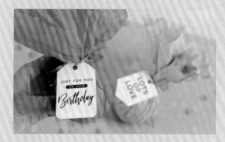

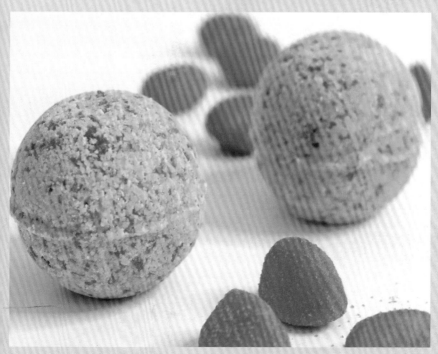

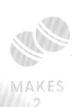

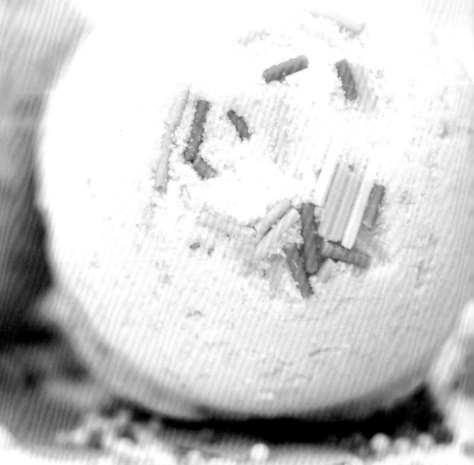

BIRTHDAY
CAKE

BIRTHDAY CAKE

This fun bath bomb is the perfect homemade gift for a loved one's birthday or special occasion!
Just remember ... don't eat it!

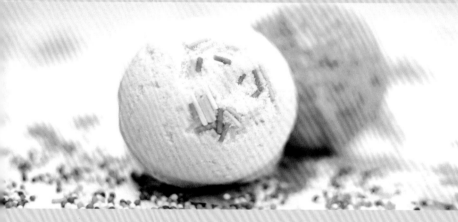

YOU WILL NEED

- A large mixing bowl
- 2 x medium mixing bowls
- Microwave
- Microwavable mug
- Whisk
- 2 x Bath Bomb moulds
- Clingfilm

INGREDIENTS

- Bicarbonate of soda 100g
- Cream of tartar 25g
- Corn starch 50g
- Epsom salt 2 tbsp
- Vanilla essential oil
  6 - 8 drops
- Green colouring 3 drops
- Coconut oil 1 – 2 tbsp
- 100s & 1000s sprinkles

METHOD

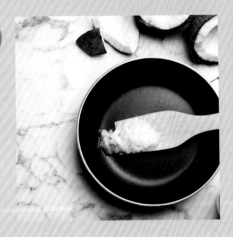

1 Always refer back to your first bath bomb and make sure you've got your work surface ready and all your equipment to hand.

2 Take your microwavable mug and add 1 – 2 tablespoons of coconut oil and 8 drops of your vanilla essential oil.

3 Microwave for 60 – 90 seconds or until the mixture is completely liquified. Make sure to only microwave 20 seconds at a time so you can check on progress. This is your oil base.

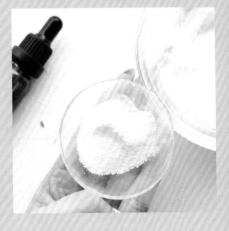

4 In your large mixing bowl, add the bicarbonate of soda, cream of tartar, corn starch and Epsom salt before mixing thoroughly.

5 Pour your liquid mixture into the dry ingredients. We suggest doing this slowly whilst whisking throughout.

6 Add a teaspoon of water to your mixture and stir again.

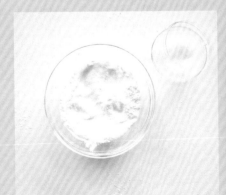

7 Once the two mixtures are combined, give it a mix with your hands to ensure it's all mixed together, you don't want any lumps.

8 You are looking for the wet sand consistency again. Refer back to the tips page for how to achieve this.

9 Separate your mix evenly into 2 bowls and add 3 drops of green colouring to one bowl and give it a good whisk.

10 Add a generous sprinkle of 100s and 1000s to one half of your bath bomb mould. We recommend a thin layer across the bottom of the mould.

11 Now pour the white mixture into the mould with the 100s & 1000s.

12 Take your other mould and fill it with the green mixture.

13 Place your moulds together and hold for 10 - 15 seconds. Wrap in clingfilm and leave overnight.

14 The next day, you can remove the bath bomb from the mould but be gentle with it. Make sure you store the bath bomb with the 100s and 1000s on the top.

TIP

When you're ready to gift the bath bomb, wrap it in coloured tissue paper and ribbon. Or why not make a few in different colours and add them to a gift box along with some shredded paper.

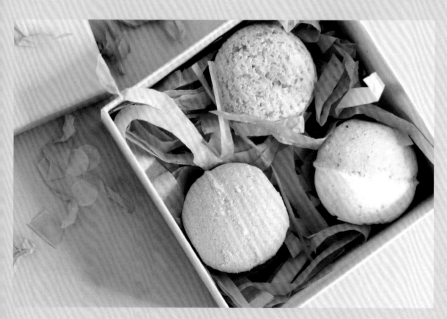

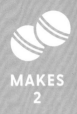

MAKES
2

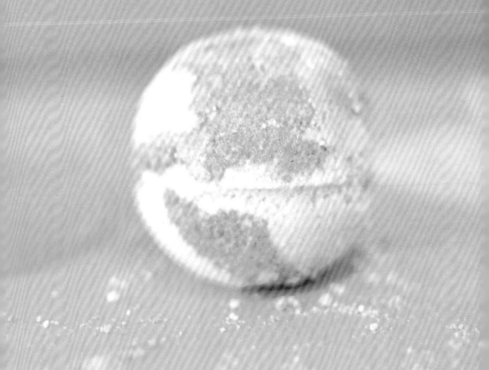

STRAWBERRIES
& CREAM

STRAWBERRIES & CREAM

Strawberries & cream - Not just for the tennis. These bath bombs will transport you back to a warm summers day.

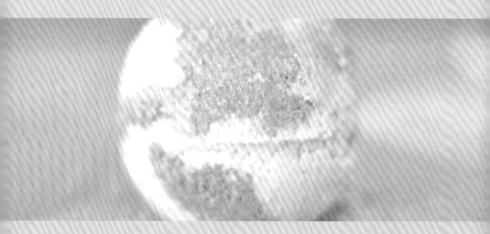

YOU WILL NEED

- A large mixing bowl
- 2 x medium mixing bowls
- Microwave
- Microwavable mug
- Whisk
- 2 x Bath Bomb moulds
- Clingfilm

INGREDIENTS

- Bicarbonate of soda 100g
- Cream of tartar 25g
- Corn starch 50g
- Epsom salt 2 tbsp
- Strawberry essential oil 6 - 8 drops
- Red colouring 10 drops
- Coconut oil 1 – 2 tbsp

METHOD

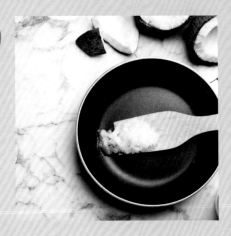

1 Always refer back to your first bath bomb and make sure you've got your work surface ready and all your equipment to hand.

2 Take your microwavable mug and add 1 – 2 tablespoons of coconut oil and 6-8 drops of your strawberry essential oil.

3 Microwave for 60 – 90 seconds or until the mixture is completely liquified. Make sure to only microwave 20 seconds at a time so you can check on progress. This is your oil base.

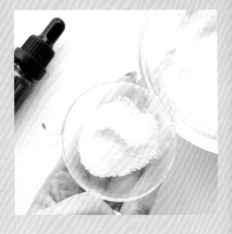

4 In your large mixing bowl, add the bicarbonate of soda, cream of tartar, corn starch and Epsom salt before mixing thoroughly.

5 Pour your liquid mixture into the dry ingredients. We suggest doing this slowly whilst whisking throughout.

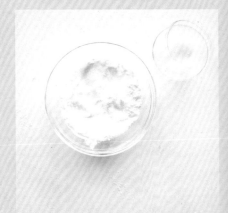

6 Add a teaspoon of water to your mixture and stir again.

7 Once the two mixtures are combined, give it a mix with your hands to ensure it's all mixed together.

8 Separate your mix evenly into 2 bowls and add 10 drops of red colouring to one bowl before giving it a good whisk.

9 Take one of your moulds and place a large pinch of the red mixture, in the mould in a spiral shape. Then use your finger to make the lines more defined and create a ripple effect.

10 Now add a sprinkle of white on top, and then red. Repeat this process until the mould half is full.

11 Take your other mould and repeat step 9 to create the strawberries and cream effect.

12 Place your moulds together and hold for 10 - 15 seconds. Wrap in clingfilm and leave overnight.

13 The next day, you can remove the bath bomb from the mould and it's ready to enjoy.

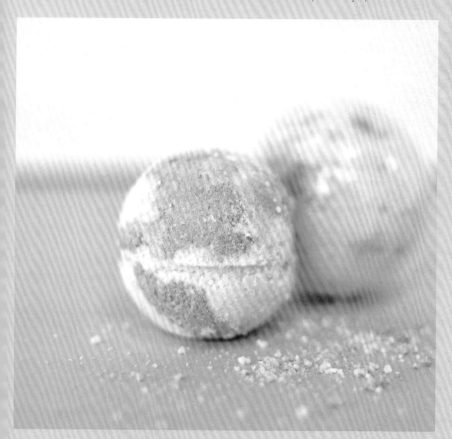

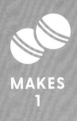

MAKES
1

LOVE HEART

LOVE HEART BATH BOMB

The perfect way to say 'I love you'. Our big heart bath bomb is guaranteed to put a smile on a loved ones face.

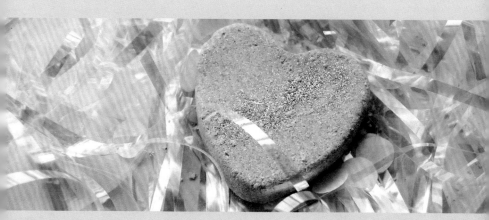

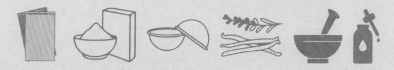

YOU WILL NEED

· A mixing bowl
· Microwave
· Microwavable mug
· Whisk
· 1 x Large heart mould
  You can try the same recipe
  with smaller hearts too!
· Clingfilm

INGREDIENTS

· Bicarbonate of soda 100g
· Cream of tartar 25g
· Corn starch 50g
· Epsom salt 2 tbsp
· Essential oil 8 drops
· Pink colouring 10-15 drops
· Coconut oil 1 – 2 tbsp
· Biodegradable glitter

METHOD

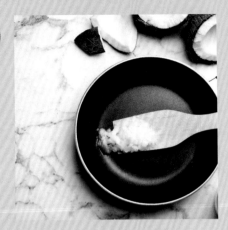

1 Always refer back to your first bath bomb and make sure you've got your work surface ready and all your equipment to hand.

2 Take your microwavable mug and add 2 tablespoons of coconut oil, 5 - 7 drops of pink colouring and 8 drops of your chosen essential oil.

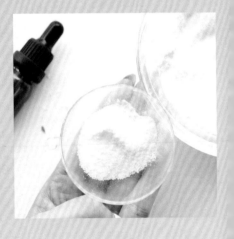

3 Microwave for 60 – 90 seconds or until the mixture is completely liquified. Make sure to only microwave 20 seconds at a time so you can check on progress. This is your oil base.

4 In your large mixing bowl, add the bicarbonate of soda, cream of tartar, corn starch and Epsom salt before mixing thoroughly.

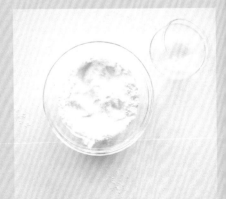

5 Pour your liquid mixture into the dry ingredients. We suggest doing this slowly whilst whisking throughout.

6 Add a teaspoon of water to your mixture and stir again.

7 Once the two mixtures are combined, give it a mix with your hands to ensure it's all mixed together.

8 If you're adding bio-degradable glitter, add it now! Take a pinch of your glitter and sprinkle it ,across the bottom of your mould.

9 Start to compact your bath bomb mould, over-packing it and using your fingers to press down the mixture, especially round the curves of the heart.

TIP

Smaller hearts for a Jar!

10 If you're using a large heart mould, place the mould upside down and push hard so the mixture comes out onto your flat surface (do this as close to the surface as possible to avoid it dropping it from a distance).

If you're using the mould included in the kit, continue to follow the method from the previous bath bombs.

11 Leave your finished bath bombs for 24 hours to dry on a flat surface.

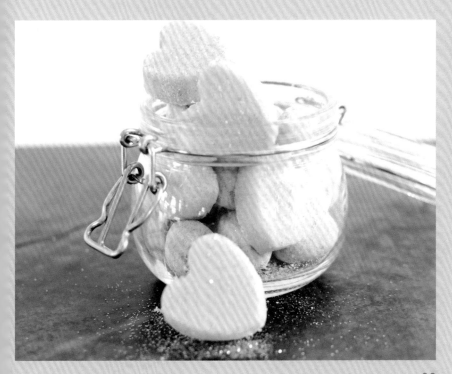

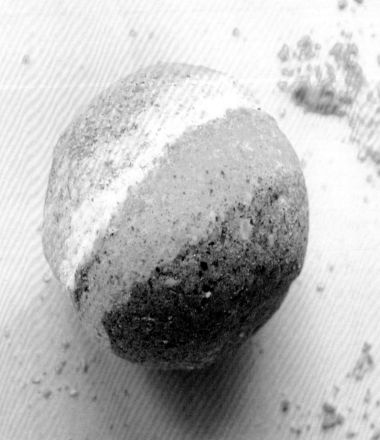

RAINBOW

RAINBOW

What better way to lift your spirits and add some colour to your bath routine. Our rainbow themed bath bomb is guaranteed to bring some excitement to bath time.

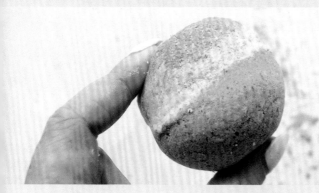

YOU WILL NEED

· A large mixing bowl
· 6 medium sized bowls
· Microwave
· Microwavable mug
· Whisk
· 2 x bath bomb moulds
· Cling film

INGREDIENTS

· Bicarbonate of soda 100g
· Cream of tartar 25g
· Corn starch 50g
· Epsom salt 2 tbsp
· Essential oil: 6-8 drops
· Coconut oil: 1 – 2 tbsp
· Pink colouring: 6 drops
· Orange colouring: 6 drops
· Yellow colouring: 6 drops
· Green colouring: 6 drops
· Blue colouring: 6 drops
· Purple colouring: 6 drops

METHOD

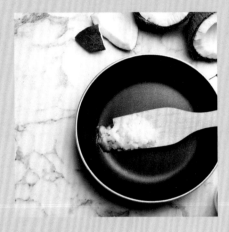

1 Take your microwavable mug and add 2 tablespoons of coconut oil and 8 drops of your chosen essential oil.

2 Microwave for 60 – 90 seconds or until the mixture is completely liquified. Make sure to only microwave 20 seconds at a time so you can check on progress. This is your oil base.

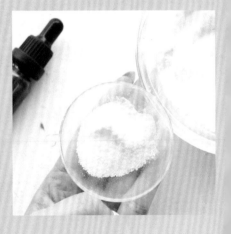

3 In your large mixing bowl add the bicarbonate of soda, cream of tartar, corn starch and Epsom salt before mixing thoroughly.

4 Pour your liquid mixture into the dry ingredients. We suggest doing this slowly whilst whisking throughout.

5 Add a teaspoon of water to your mixture and stir again.

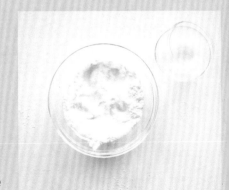

6 Once the two mixtures are combined, give it a mix with your hands to ensure it's all mixed together. Remember it's the wet sand consistency you're looking for!

7 Separate your mix evenly across 6 bowls and add 6 drops of colouring to each bowl before whisking well. Each bowl should be a different colour.

8 Take one of your moulds and add a large pinch of the purple mixture. You want to fill a third of the mould half and make sure it's flat.

9 Repeat this step again with the blue mixture, followed by the green mixture. Make sure it is tightly compacted.

10 Take your other mould half and grab a large pinch of the pink mixture, again enough to fill a third of the mould.

11 Repeat this step again with the orange mixture, followed by the yellow mixture, compacting like your first mould.

12 Press them together as you have in previous bath bomb projects and wrap in cling film. Leave overnight to dry.

13 The next day, you can remove the bath bomb from the mould and it's ready to enjoy!

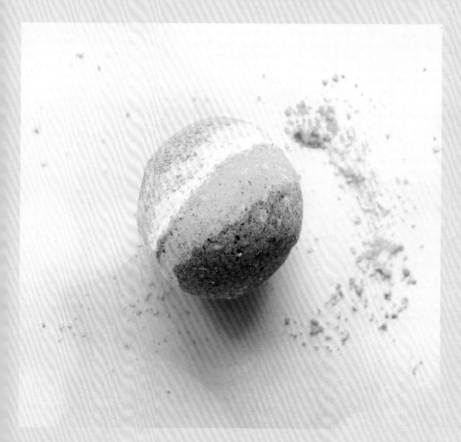

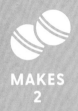

MAKES
2

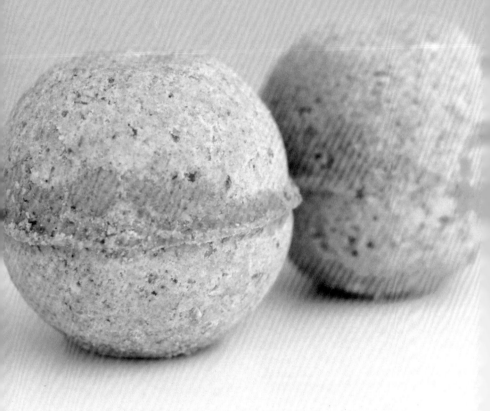

MERMAID

MERMAID

With this bath bomb, you'll feel like you're swimming with mermaids. These wonderful colours will create the ideal setting for your bath.

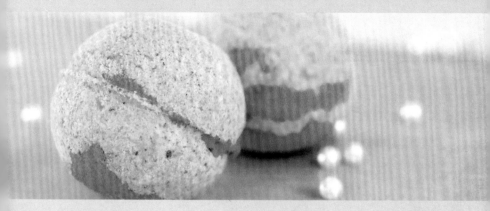

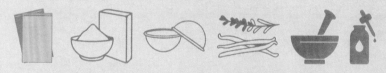

YOU WILL NEED

· A mixing bowl
· 3 x small mixing bowls
· Microwave
· Microwavable mug
· Whisk
· 2 x Bath Bomb moulds
· Clingfilm

INGREDIENTS

· Bicarbonate of soda 100g
· Cream of tartar 25g
· Corn starch 50g
· Epsom salt 2 tbsp
· Essential oil: 6-8 drops
· Coconut oil: 1 – 2 tbsp
· Pink colouring : 6 drops
· Purple colouring: 3 drops
· Green colouring: 4 drops

METHOD

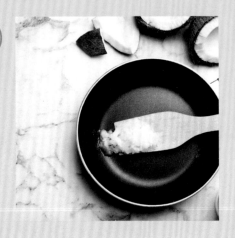

1 Take your microwavable mug and add 2 tablespoons of coconut oil and 8 drops of your chosen essential oil.

2 Microwave for 60 – 90 seconds or until the mixture is completely liquified. Make sure to only microwave 20 seconds at a time so you can check on progress. This is your oil base.

3 In your large mixing bowl add the bicarbonate of soda, cream of tartar, corn starch and Epsom salt before mixing thoroughly.

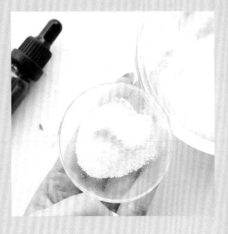

4 Pour your liquid mixture into the dry ingredients. We suggest doing this slowly whilst whisking throughout.

5 Add a teaspoon of water to your mixture and stir again.

6 Once the two mixtures are combined, give it a mix with your hands to ensure it's all mixed together. Remember it's the wet sand consistency you're looking for!

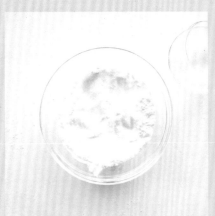

7 Separate your mix into 3 bowls, 1 bowl having 50% of the mixture and the other two bowls having 25% each.

8 Add 6 drops of pink colouring to the bowl with 50% of mixture.

9 Add 4 drops of green colouring to the second bowl and 4 drops of purple colouring to the third bowl.

10 Give the coloured mixes a stir and add colouring until you're happy with the colour. Be careful not to overdo it as this may add too much moisture to your mix.

11 Grab one of your moulds and add a pinch of the pink mixture, then unevenly add a section of the green mixture around the wall of the mould.

12 Follow with a random splash of the purple mixture. You can be as messy as you want with this step to create a wavey look.

13 Once you reach the rim of the mould, grab a large handful of the pink mixture and overpack the mould.

14 Take the other mould and add a pinch of the green and purple mixture in the bottom. You can then freestyle between your colours until nearly full. Finish with a large pinch of pink mixture on top.

15 Place your moulds together and hold for 10 - 15 seconds. Wrap in clingfilm and leave overnight.

16 The next day, you can remove the bath bomb from the mould and it's ready to enjoy!

TIP

Put in a personalised box + matching ribbon to finish this special mermaid bath bomb gift!

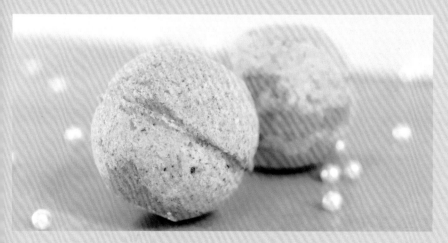

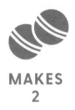

MAKES
2

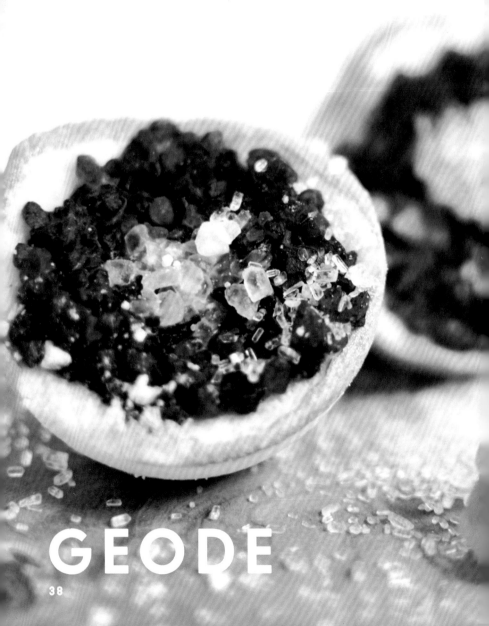

GEODE

GEODE

This crystal inspired bath bomb will add some sparkle and class to your bath time. Make bath time that bit more blingy!

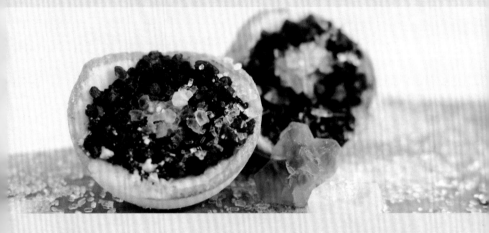

YOU WILL NEED

- A large mixing bowl
- Pipette or similar
- 1 small bowl
- A Spoon
- Microwave
- Microwavable mug
- Whisk
- 4 x Bath Bomb moulds
- Cling film
- Small container
- Small paint brush

INGREDIENTS

- Bicarbonate of soda 100g
- Cream of tartar 25g
- Corn starch 50g
- Epsom salt 1 tbsp
- Rock salt 50g
- Essential oil: 6 - 8 drops
- Coconut oil: 3 tbsp
- Purple colouring: 8 drops
- Gold mica powder
- Witch hazel

METHOD

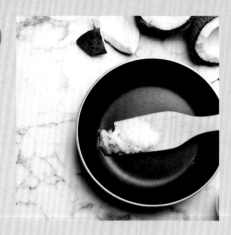

1 Take your microwavable mug and add 2 tablespoons of coconut oil and 6 – 8 drops of your chosen essential oil.

2 Microwave for 60 – 90 seconds or until the mixture is completely liquified. Make sure to only microwave 20 seconds at a time so you can check on progress. This is your oil base.

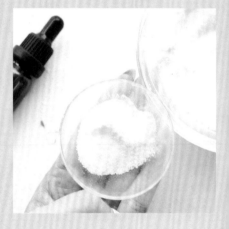

3 In your large mixing bowl add the bicarbonate of soda, cream of tartar, corn starch and Epsom salt before mixing thoroughly.

4 Pour your liquid mixture into the dry ingredients. We suggest doing this slowly whilst whisking throughout.

5 Add a teaspoon of water to your mixture and stir again.

6 Once the two mixtures are combined, give it a mix with your hands to ensure it's all mixed together. Remember it's the wet sand consistency you're looking for!

7 Take one of your moulds and add a dusting of corn starch around the mould to prevent sticking.

8 On top of the corn starch, add the bath bomb mixture until its reached the rim.

9 Using your thumbs, press the mixture firmly down to create a dipped bowl like shape in the mould.

10 Leave the mixture in the bath bomb mould on a flat surface for 24 hours.

11 The next day, give your moulds a gentle tap with a metal spoon and delicately ease the bath bomb out off the mould.
TIP: If they are struggling to come out, turn the mould over onto a flat surface and gently tap the top until you hear it drop.

12 To add that sparkly touch, you're now going to paint the rims of the bath bombs. Mix a small amount of witch hazel and gold mica powder in a small container and use a small paint brush to carefully paint the edge of the bath bomb.

13 To make the crystal topping, add 1 – 2 tablespoons of coconut oil to a microwavable mug for 60 seconds or until fully liquified.

14 Take a small bowl and add 80% of your rock salt, followed by 8 drops of purple colouring and stir well.

15 Using your pipette, spread a few drops of coconut oil into the dipped centre of your bath bomb, followed by a good heap of purple salt mixture.

16 Now take a pinch of uncoloured rock salt and sprinkle it in the very centre.

17 Carefully pipette or spoon your melted coconut oil over the salts, making sure to cover all of them but be careful not to flood them.

18 Leave your geode bath bombs to dry on a flat surface for 6-8 hours before wrapping up or using.

TIP
This is a perfect spa gift!

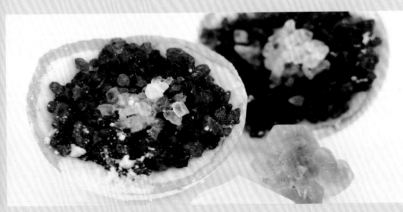

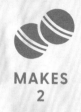

**MAKES
2**

SUNSET

SUNSET

Everybody loves a sunset so why not recreate your very own perfect end to the day. Gift someone a little ray of sunshine with this vibrant bath bomb!

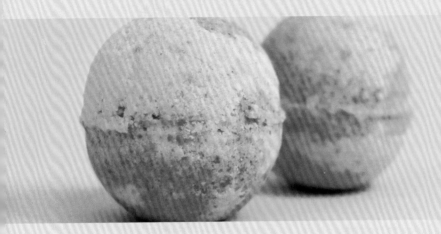

YOU WILL NEED

- A mixing bowl
- Microwave
- Microwavable mug
- Whisk
- 2 x Bath Bomb moulds
- Clingfilm

INGREDIENTS

- Bicarbonate of soda 100g
- Cream of tartar 25g
- Corn starch 50g
- Epsom salt 2 tbsp
- Sweet orange essential oil: 6-8 drops
- Coconut oil: 1 – 2 tbsp
- Orange colouring: 8-10 drops
- Yellow colouring: 8-10 drops

METHOD

1 Take your microwavable mug and add 2 tablespoons of coconut oil and 6 – 8 drops of the sweet orange essential oil.

2 Microwave for 60 – 90 seconds or until the mixture is completely liquified. Make sure to only microwave 20 seconds at a time so you can check on progress. This is your oil base.

3 In your large mixing bowl add the bicarbonate of soda, cream of tartar, corn starch and Epsom salt before mixing thoroughly.

4 Pour your liquid mixture into the dry ingredients. We suggest doing this slowly whilst whisking throughout.

5 Add a teaspoon of water to your mixture and stir again.

6 Once the two mixtures are combined, give it a mix with your hands to ensure it's all mixed together. Remember it's the wet sand consistency you're looking for. Divide your mix into 2 bowls.

8 Add 8-10 drops of orange colouring to one bowl, and 8-10 drops of yellow to the other.

9 Take one of your moulds and drop in a small amount of orange mixture. Use your finger to create uneven shaped empty areas,

10 Drop a large pinch of the yellow mix on top and keep unevenly stacking the colours until the mould is full.

11 Take the other mould and this time, add a larger pinch of orange mix to the bottom of the mould and flatten it out.

12 Fill the rest of the mould up with uneven heaps of the 2 colours until full.

13 Place your moulds together and hold for 10 - 15 seconds. Wrap in clingfilm and leave overnight.

14 The next day, you can remove the bath bomb from the mould and it's ready to enjoy!

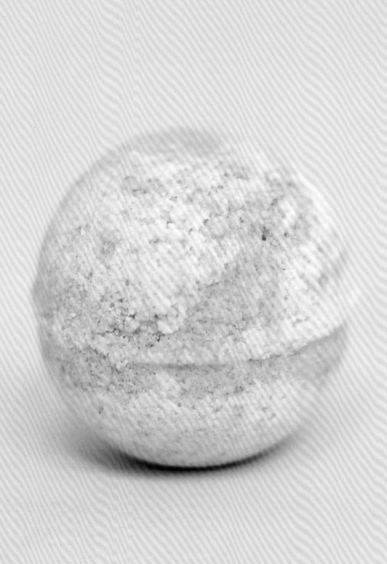

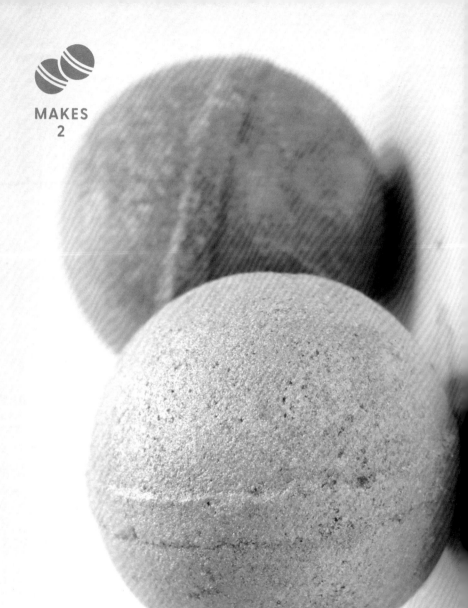

SHIMMER

SHIMMER

There's nothing better than a bit of glitz and glam which is why the shimmer bath bomb is the perfect accompaniment to your bath routine.

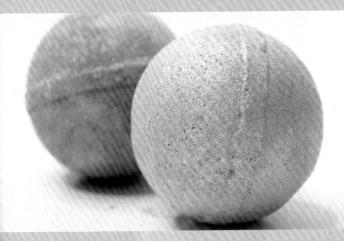

YOU WILL NEED

· A mixing bowl
· Microwave
· Microwavable mug
· Whisk
· 2 x bath bomb moulds
· Cling film

INGREDIENTS

· Bicarbonate of soda 100g
· Cream of tartar 25g
· Corn starch 50g
· Epsom salt 2 tbsp
· Essential oil 6 - 8 drops
· Blue colouring 10 - 15 drops
· Coconut oil 1 – 2 tbsp
· Spray glitter colours
  (like the ones used for
  cakes)

METHOD

1 Always refer back to your first bath bomb and make sure you've got your work surface ready and all your equipment to hand.

2 Take your microwavable mug and add 1 – 2 tablespoons of coconut oil, 10 drops of blue colouring and 6 – 8 drops of your chosen essential oil.

3 Microwave for 60 – 90 seconds or until the mixture is completely liquified. Make sure to only microwave 20 seconds at a time so you can check on progress. This is your oil base.

4 In your mixing bowl, add the bicarbonate of soda, cream of tartar, corn starch and Epsom salt before mixing thoroughly.

5 Pour your liquid mixture into the dry ingredients. We suggest doing this slowly whilst whisking throughout.

6 Add a teaspoon of water to your mixture and stir again.

7 Once the two mixtures are combined, give it a mix with your hands to ensure it's all mixed together (you don't want any lumps).

8 You are looking for the wet sand consistency again. If you think it is too dry then add half a teaspoon of water and mix again. If you feel it's too wet then add a couple of teaspoons of bicarbonate of soda.

9 Start to compact your bath bomb moulds and fill again just above the rim - the same as you did in your first project.

10 Place your moulds together and hold for 10 - 15 seconds. Wrap in clingfilm and leave overnight.

11 The next day, remove your bath bomb and place on a surface suitable for spraying.

12 Take your first colour of spray glitter and spray one half of your bath bomb.

13 Grab your second spray bottle and spray a quarter of the side you have already sprayed, to create a gradient effect.

14 Leave to dry for 24 hours before spraying the other side the same way to ensure an even effect.

Horse Yoga

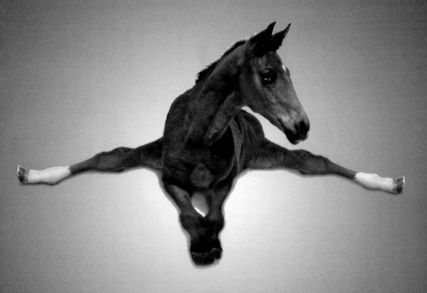

RAVETTE PUBLISHING

First published by Ravette Publishing 2017

Ravette Publishing Limited
PO Box 876
Horsham
West Sussex RH12 9GH

ISBN: 978-1-84161-401-4
Printed and bound in India by Replika Press Pvt. Ltd.

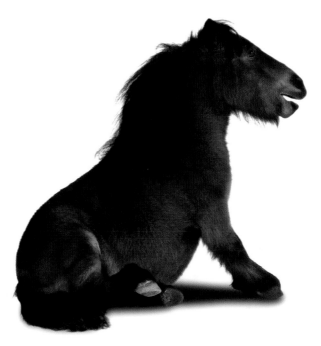

Attitude is a little thing
that makes a big difference.

Winston Churchill

My point is,
life is about balance.
The good and the bad.
The highs and the lows.
The pina and the colada.

Ellen DeGeneres

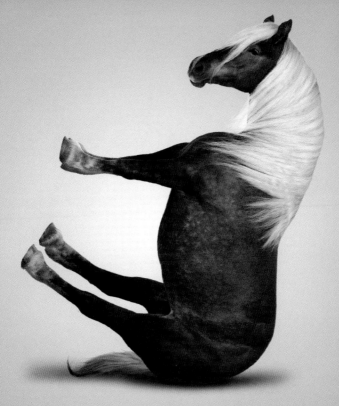

BALANCE

Courage isn't having the strength to go on – it is going on when you don't have strength.

Napoléon Bonaparte

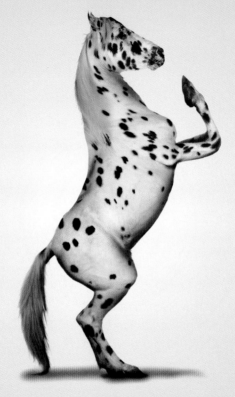

COURAGE

Determine that the thing can and shall be done and then ... find the way.

Abraham Lincoln

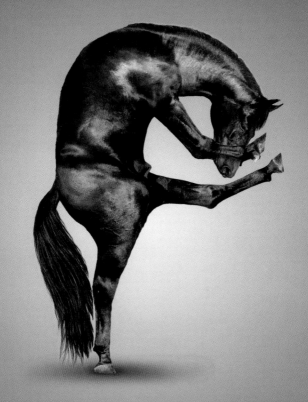

DETERMINATION

Happiness
is good health and
a bad memory.

Ingrid Bergman

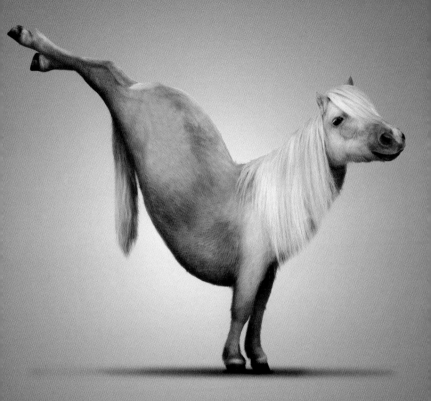

HAPPINESS

To put everything in
balance is good,
to put everything in
harmony is better.

Victor Hugo

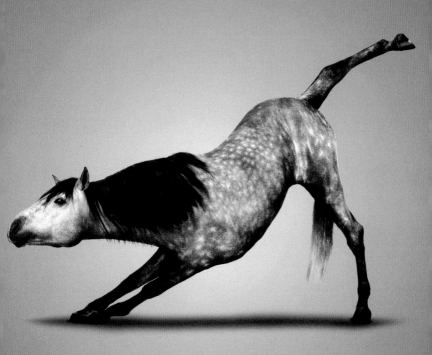

HARMONY

Kindness is a language which the deaf can hear and the blind can see.

Mark Twain

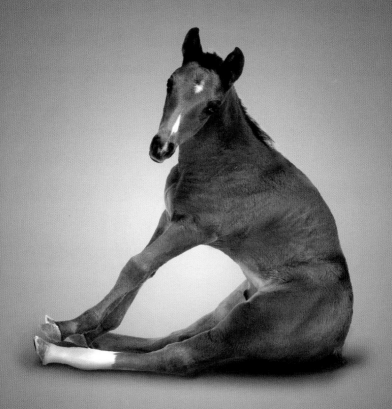

KINDNESS

Nothing great in the world was accomplished without passion.

Georg Wilhelm Friedrich Hegel

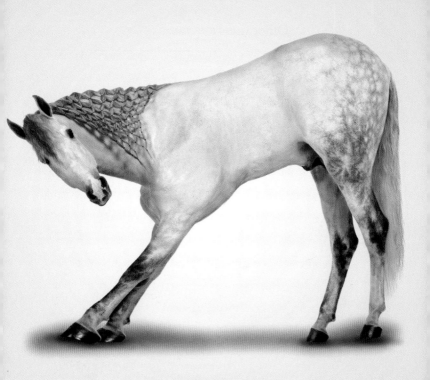

PASSION

Patience is bitter,
but its fruit
is sweet.

Aristotle

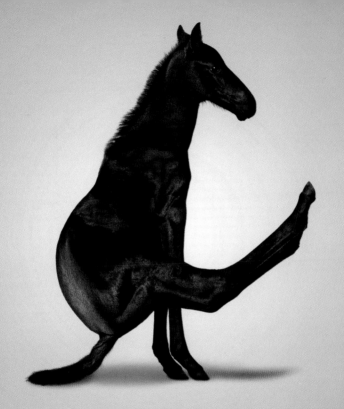

PATIENCE

You cannot find peace
by avoiding life.

Virginia Woolf

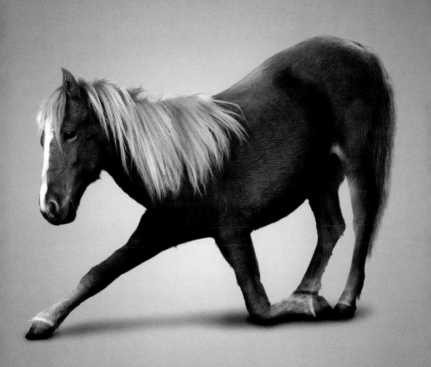

PEACE

Enthusiasm
is a supernatural
serenity.

Henry David Thoreau

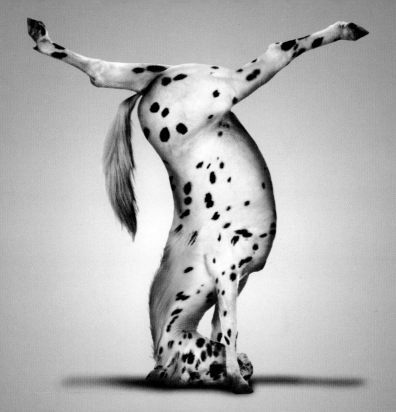

SERENITY

You have power
over your mind
– not outside events.
Realise this and you will
find strength.

Marcus Aurelius

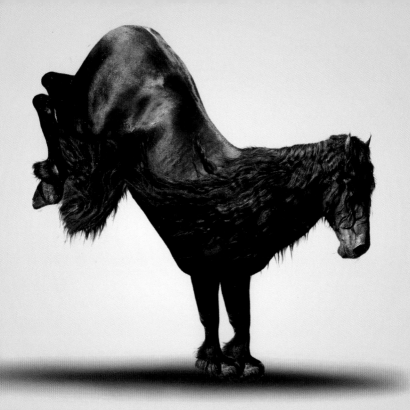

STRENGTH

What divides us
pales in comparison
to what unites us.

Edward Kennedy

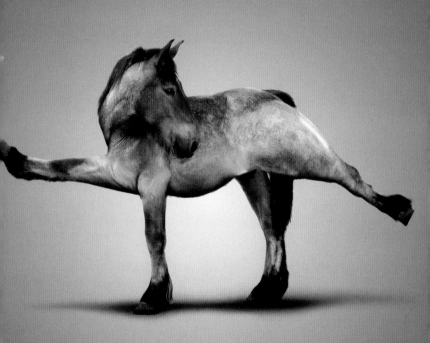

UNITY

The best fighter
is never angry.

Lao Tzu

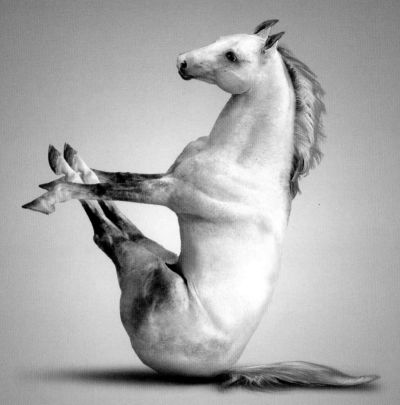

WARRIOR

Wisdom is not a product of schooling, but of the lifelong attempt to acquire it.

Albert Einstein

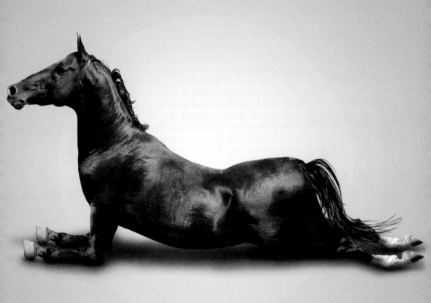

WISDOM

Other titles available in this series ...

	ISBN	Price
Animal Yoga	978-1-84161-390-1	£5.99
Cow Yoga	978-1-84161-389-5	£5.99
Farmyard Yoga	978-1-84161-396-3	£5.99

How to order   Please send a cheque/postal order in £ sterling, made payable
to 'Ravette Publishing' for the cover price of the book/s and
allow the following for post & packaging ...

UK & BFPO   70p for the first book & 40p per book thereafter
Europe and Eire   £1.30 for the first book & 70p per book thereafter
Rest of the world £2.20 for the first book & £1.10 per book thereafter

RAVETTE PUBLISHING LTD
PO Box 876, Horsham, West Sussex RH12 9GH
Tel: 01403 711443   Email: info@ravettepub.co.uk
www.ravettepublishing.tel

Prices and availability are subject to change without prior notice.